Recipes for a Mediterranean Diet

How to Cook Mediterranean Style

Debbie G. Byrd

Contents

Chapter One

INTRODUCTION

Recipes for a Mediterranean Diet

How to Cook Mediterranean Style

Author

Debbie G. Byrd

The Mediterranean diet has become a well-known option for those who want to get the benefits of today's plant-based foods. The eating plan has attracted the attention of logical experts and scientists from all across the globe. Many studies have been conducted to better understand the benefits that may be associated with a Mediterranean diet.

People who follow a Mediterranean diet have been proven to have a reduced risk of coronary artery disease, aggravation, and weight loss. Glucose levels seem to be controlled as well by following this diet.

Preparing meals that are suitable for a Mediterranean diet might take some time from time to time. As a result, it's not uncommon to see people who follow this particular diet use a pressure cooker or a moment pot. These tools make preparing suppers a lot easier and faster. Simultaneously, they provide extra advantages to those who adopt a Mediterranean diet.

In this article, we'll look at what the Mediterranean diet entails. We also look at the dietary regimen's historical background. The article discusses the multiple health benefits that have been linked to eating habits. We also consider the benefits of using a pressure cooker or instant pot to prepare meals while adhering to the Mediterranean diet.

Chapter Two

The Mediterranean Diet's Origins

The Mediterranean diet is based on nutritional trends from several cultures. A few of groups were initially in charge of disseminating the eating pattern. Ancel Keys, a scientist, and Markaret Keys, a physicist, collaborated to develop an eating regimen that focuses on combining multiple food patterns into a single eating routine. It was presented for the first time in 1975.

The diet is based on nutritional patterns seen in Italy and Greece. In the 1960s, the Mediterranean eating regimen's nutritional patterns were immensely popular in these two countries.

What is the Mediterranean Diet and why is it so popular? The Mediterranean diet focuses on teaching us how to include more fresh veggies and natural items into our diets, while still providing all of the essential nutrients and minerals that our bodies need. Keeping in mind that red meat should only be consumed on rare occasions, fish and fish are a must-have. Eggs, yogurt, milk, and cheddar are also welcome, but only in moderation. Desserts, artificial sweeteners, handled meat, and highly processed food sources have no place in the Mediterranean diet.

Numerous health advantages have been linked to the Mediterranean diet.

Cardiovascular health has improved

Reduced chances of becoming sick and having a heart attack.

Low levels of cholesterol

Hypertension risk is reduced.

Stroke risk is reduced.

Diabetes mellitus risk is reduced, and the disease is progressing.

Diabetes mellitus is a kind of diabetes that affects people of all ages.

Loss of weight

Reduced facial kinks and dingy skin areas

RECIPES FOR POULTRY 1– CHICKEN FOR FAMILY DINNER

6 people

Time to prepare: 25 minutes Time to prepare: 15 minutes

Ingredients:

2 tbsp. extra virgin olive oil

a teaspoon of garlic powder

1 tablespoon paprika

To taste, season with salt and freshly ground dark pepper.

1 entire chicken (212 lb.) with neck and giblets removed

1 lemon, quartered into four wedges

1 quart of chicken broth

Instructions:) In a little bowl, combine as one the oil, flavors, salt and dark pepper.) Insert lemon wedges inside the pit of chicken.) Coat the top piece of chicken with oil combination generously.) Select "Sauté" of Instant Pot. Then, at that point, place the chicken,

bosom side down and cook for around 3-4 minutes.) Now, cover the base side of the chicken with residual flavor mixture.) Flip the chicken and cook for around 1 moment more.

) Select "Drop" and move the chicken onto a plate.

) Now, orchestrate the trivet in the lower part of Instant Pot and pour the broth.) Place the chicken on top of trivet, bosom side down.

0

) Secure the top and spot the strain valve to"Seal" position. 1) Select "Manual" and cook under "High Pressure" for around 20 minutes. 2) Select "Drop" and do a "Whiz" release.

Remove the top and spot chicken onto a cutting load up for around

10 minutes before carving.

With a sharp blade, cut chicken into wants estimated pieces and serve. Nutrition Information:

Calories per serving: 409; Carbohydrates: 0.9g; Protein: 55.7g; Fat: 19g; Sugar: 0.3g; Sodium: 317mg; Fiber: 0.3g

2– Popular Chicken Cacciatore

Serves: 4

Cooking Time: 30 minutes Preparation Time: 15

minutes

Ingredients:

2 tbsp. extra-virgin olive oil

4 (6-oz.) bone-in, skin-on chicken thighs

1 (4-oz.) bundle cut new mushrooms

3 celery stems, chopped ½ of onion, chopped

2 garlic cloves, minced

1 (14-oz.) can stewed tomatoes

2 tbsp. tomato paste

2 tsp. Herbes de Provence

3 chicken bouillon shapes, crumbled ¾ C. water

Pinch of red pepper flakes

Freshly ground dark pepper, to taste

Instructions:) Place the oil in Instant Pot and select"Sauté". Then, at that point, add the chicken thighs and cook for around 5-6 minutes for every side.

) With an opened spoon, move chicken thighs onto a plate.

) In the pot, add the mushrooms, celery and onion and cook for around 5 minutes.) Add the garlic and cook for around 2 minutes.

) Select "Drop" and mix in the chicken, tomatoes, tomato glue, Herbes de Provence, bouillon 3D shapes and water.

) Secure the cover and spot the tension valve to"Seal" position.

) Select "Manual" and cook under "High Pressure" for around 11 minutes.

) Select "Drop" and cautiously do a"Speedy" release.

) Remove the cover and mix in red pepper chips and dark pepper.

Nutrition Information: Calories per serving: 430; Carbohydrates: 9.2g; Protein: 52.1g; Fat: 20.2g; Sugar: 5.3g; Sodium: 631mg; Fiber: 2.4g

3– Famous Chicken Piccata

Serves: 4

Cooking Time: 16 minutes Time to prepare: 15 minutes

Ingredients: 4 (6-oz.) skinless, boneless chicken breasts

To taste, season with salt and freshly ground dark pepper.

1 tbsp. extra-virgin olive oil

1 C. low-sodium chicken broth ¼ C. new lemon juice

2 tbsp. cold butter

2 tbsp. tenderized escapades, drained

2 tbsp. new parsley, chopped

Instructions:) Season the chicken bosoms with salt and dark pepper evenly.) Place the oil in Instant Pot and select"Sauté". Then, at that point, add

the chicken and cook for around 2-3 minutes for every side.) Select "Drop" and pour in the broth.

) Secure the top and spot the tension valve to"Seal" position.) Select "Manual" and cook under "High Pressure" for around 3 minutes.) Select "Drop" and cautiously do a"Speedy" release.

) Remove the top and with utensils, move the chicken bosoms onto a

serving platter.) With a piece of foil, cover the chicken bosoms to keep warm.) Select "Sauté" of Instant Pot and mix in the lemon juice.

Cook for around 5-7 minutes.

Select "Drop" and include the spread, beating continuously. 2) Stir in the tricks and parsley and pour the sauce over chicken. 3) Serve immediately.

Nutrition Information:

Calories per serving: 303; Carbohydrates: 0.9g; Protein: 38.8g; Fat: 15.5g; Sugar: 0.4g; Sodium: 289mg; Fiber: 0.3g

4– Flavorsome Caprese Chicken

6 people

Cooking Time: 15 minutes Time to prepare: 15 minutes

Ingredients: ¼ C. chicken broth ¼ C. balsamic vinegar ¼ C. maple syrup

6 (4-oz.) boneless, skinless chicken breasts

8 mozzarella cheddar slices

3 C. cherry tomatoes, halved ½ C. new basil leaves, torn

Instructions:

) In the pot of Instant Pot, place the stock, vinegar and maple syrup and mix to combine.

) Add the chicken bosoms and mix to combine.

) Secure the cover and spot the tension valve to"Seal" position.) Select "Manual" and cook under "High Pressure" for around 8 minutes.) Meanwhile, preheat the stove to broiler.

) Select "Drop" and cautiously do a"Speedy" release.

) Remove the top of Instant pot and with an opened spoon, move

the chicken bosoms onto a baking sheet.) Place a cut of cheddar on every chicken breast.) Select "Sauté" of Instant Pot and cook for around 4-5 minutes. 0) Stir in the tomatoes and cook for around 1-2 minutes.

Stir in the basil and select "Cancel".

Meanwhile, sear the chicken bosoms for around 2-3 minutes or until

cheddar is melted.

Divide the chicken bosoms onto serving plates and present with the garnish of tomato sauce.

Nutrition Information:

Calories per serving: 377; Carbohydrates: 13.8g; Protein: 54.7g; Fat: 15.4g; Sugar: 10.3g; Sodium: 362mg; Fiber: 1.1g

5– Purely Greek Flavored Chicken Serves: 8

Cooking Time: 18 minutes Time to prepare: 15 minutes
Ingredients:

1 tbsp. garlic and spice seasoning

½ tsp. garlic salt ¼ tsp. ground dark pepper

2 lb. skinless, boneless chicken breasts

2 tbsp. avocado oil

6 simmered garlic cloves, mashed

1 (8 oz.) container marinated artichoke hearts, drained

1 C. cut Kalamata olives

½ of medium red onion, sliced ½ of (16 liquid oz.) bottle Greek serving of mixed greens dressing   1 tbsp. arrowroot starch

1 (4-oz.) bundle feta cheddar, crumbled

Instructions:

) In a bowl, combine as one the garlic and spice preparing, garlic salt, and dark pepper.) Season every chicken bosom with preparing combination evenly.

) Place the oil in Instant Pot and select"Sauté". Then, at that point, add the garlic and cook for around 1 minute.) Place the chicken bosoms and cook for around 2 minutes for every side.

) Select "Drop" and spot the artichoke hearts and olives around and top of the chicken breasts.

) Top with onion, trailed by dressing.

) Secure the cover and spot the strain valve to"Seal" position.
) Select "Manual" and cook under "High Pressure" for around 15 minutes.) Select "Drop" and cautiously do a"Fast" release.

Remove the top of Instant pot and with an opened spoon, move the chicken bosoms onto a plate.

In the pot, add the arrowroot starch and thump until well combined.

Stir in the cooked chicken and select"Sauté".

Cook for around 3 minutes.

Select "Drop" and serve hot with the garnish of feta cheese. Nutrition Information: Calories per serving: 406; Carbohydrates: 8.2g; Protein: 28.7g; Fat: 29.3g; Sugar: 1.2g; Sodium: 572mg; Fiber: 2.5g

6– Braised Chicken Serves: 4

Cooking Time: 18 minutes Time to prepare: 15 minutes Ingredients:

8 (4-oz.) skinless, boneless chicken thighs

Salt, to taste

2 tbsp. extra virgin olive oil

2 oz. pancetta, chopped ½ of huge red onion, sliced 2 garlic cloves, chopped ½ C. dry white wine

1 C. red peppers, cultivated and sliced

1 C. cut cured simmered peppers

2 new rosemary sprigs

2 tbsp. balsamic vinegar

2 tbsp. new lemon juice

1 oz. butter

Instructions:) Season the chicken thighs with salt equally and set aside.) Place the oil in Instant Pot and select"Sauté". Then, at that point, add 4

chicken thighs and cook for around 1-2 minutes for each side.) With an opened spoon, move the chicken thighs onto a plate.) Repeat with the leftover chicken thighs.))

2 minutes.

) Add the wine and cook for around 1 moment, scraping up the carmelized bits from the bottom.) Select "Drop" and mix in the excess fixings with the exception of butter.) Place the cooked chicken thighs on top and tenderly, cover with some of onions and peppers. Secure the cover and spot the tension valve to

"Seal" position.) Select "Manual" and cook under "High Pressure" for around 10 minutes. 0) Select "Drop" and cautiously do a"Fast" release.

1) Remove the top and with an opened spoon, move the chicken thighs onto a plate.

Select "Sauté" and cook for around 5 minutes.

Add the spread and mix until dissolved completely.

Select "Drop" and pour the sauce over chicken thighs.

Serve immediately.

Nutrition Information:

Calories per serving: 539; Carbohydrates: 10.1g; Protein: 57.7g; Fat: 27.2g; Sugar: 5.2g; Sodium: 499mg; Fiber: 1.6g

7– Moroccan Chicken Meal Serves: 6

Cooking Time: 20 minutes Time to prepare: 15 minutes

Ingredients:

1 tbsp. oil

2 lb. boneless chicken thighs, managed and cut into huge chunks   2 red peppers, cut into chunks

1 enormous onion

4 garlic cloves

2 Roma tomatoes, cut into chunks

1 (15-oz.) can chickpeas, washed and drained

1 tsp. salt ½ tsp. newly ground dark pepper

1 tsp. ground cumin ½ tsp. ground coriander

1 tsp. dried parsley

½ tsp. za'atar

1 C. tomato sauce

Instructions:

) Place the oil in Instant Pot and select"Sauté". Then, at that point, add the onion and garlic and cook for around 5 minutes.) Add the chicken lumps, and cook for around 3-5 minutes or carmelized from all sides.

) Select "Drop" and mix in the excess ingredients.

) Secure the cover and spot the tension valve to"Seal" position.) Select "Manual" and cook under "High Pressure" for around 10 minutes.

) Select "Drop" and cautiously do a"Fast" release.) Remove the top and serve hot. Nutrition Information:

Calories per serving: 430; Carbohydrates: 24.4g; Protein: 48.9g; Fat: 14.6g; Sugar: 4.7g; Sodium: 949mg; Fiber: 5.1g

14– 2-Cheeses Chicken Serves: 4

Cooking Time: 10 minutes Time to prepare: 15 minutes

Ingredients: 4 (6 oz.) boneless, skinless chicken bosom halves

1 (14½-oz.) can diced tomatoes with juices

1 (12-oz.) container marinated quartered artichoke hearts, undrained   2 tsp. Italian seasoning

¾ tsp. garlic salt

1 C. mozzarella cheddar, shredded ¼ C. Parmesan cheddar, grated

Instructions:

) In the pot of Instant Pot, place the chicken bosom parts and top with tomatoes, trailed by the artichokes.

) Sprinkle with Italian flavoring and garlic salt.

) Secure the top and spot the tension valve to"Seal" position.

) Select "Manual" and cook under "High Pressure" for around 10 minutes.

) Select "Drop" and do a "Whiz" discharge for around 10 minutes, then, at that point, do a "Fast" release.

) Remove the top and quickly, sprinkle the chicken combination with both cheeses.) Immediately, cover the moment pot with a top for around 5 minutes before serving.

Nutrition Information: Calories per serving: 429; Carbohydrates: 13.8g; Protein: 57g; Fat: 16.1g; Sugar: 3.9g; Sodium: 318mg; Fiber: 5.9g

15– Low-Carb Dinner Meal Serves: 8

Cooking Time: 10 minutes Time to prepare: 15 minutes

Ingredients:

4 (8-oz.) boneless, skinless chicken bosoms, divided and beat thinly   4 garlic cloves, minced 1 tbsp. Italian flavoring blend

Salt, to taste

2 tbsp. extra-virgin olive oil

2 tbsp. butter

¾ C. weighty whipping cream

¼ C. low-sodium chicken broth

1 tsp. prepared salt

¾ C. Parmigiano-Reggiano cheese

½ C. sun-dried tomatoes

2 C. new spinach

Instructions:

) In a huge bowl, add the chicken bosoms, garlic, Italian flavoring and salt and blend well.) Place the oil and margarine in Instant Pot and select "Sauté". Then, at that point, add the chicken bosoms and cook for around 1 moment for every side.

) Select "Drop" and mix in the cream, stock and prepared salt

) Secure the top and spot the tension valve to"Seal" position.) Select "Manual" and cook under "High Pressure" for around 1 minute.

) Select "Drop" and do a "Whiz" discharge for around 4 minutes, then, at that point, do a "Speedy" release.) Remove the top and mix the blend well.) Select "Sauté" and bring to a delicate simmer.) Stir in the cheddar and sun-dried tomatoes and cook for around 2-3 minutes.

Stir in the spinach and cook for around 1 minute.

Select "Drop" and serve hot.

Nutrition Information:

Calories per serving: 346; Carbohydrates: 1.6g; Protein: 36.5g; Fat: 21.3g; Sugar: 0.4g; Sodium: 386mg; Fiber: 0.3g

16– Souvlaki Inspired Chicken Bowl

Serves: 4

Cooking Time: 3 minutes Preparation Time: 20 minutes

Ingredients:

½ C. also 2 tbsp. water, divided ¼ C. also 2 tbsp. olive oil, divided 3 garlic cloves, ground and divided ½ tsp. dried oregano

½ tsp. paprika

Pinch of squashed red pepper flakes

To taste, season with salt and freshly ground dark pepper.

1½ lb. boneless, skinless chicken bosoms, cut into ½-inch thick slices   1 C. couscous

1 C. full-fat Greek yogurt

2 tbsp. new lemon juice

1 English cucumber, chopped

1 C. cherry tomatoes, quartered ½ C. Kalamata olives, pitted and chopped

½ C. feta cheddar, crumbled

2 tbsp. new dill, chopped

Instructions:) In the pot of Instant Pot, ½ C. of the water, ¼ C. of olive oil, 2 garlic cloves, oregano, paprika, red pepper pieces, salt and dark pepper and blend well.

) Add the chicken, cuts and mix to combine.

) Secure the top and spot the strain valve to"Seal" position.) Select "Manual" and cook under "High Pressure" for around 3 minutes.) Select "Drop" and cautiously do a"Fast" release.

) Remove the top and with an opened spoon, move the chicken cuts into a

bowl.) In the pot, add the couscous, salt and dark pepper and mix to combine.) With a glass top, cover the Instant Pot for around 6-7 minutes or

until couscous is delicate and fluffy.) Uncover the pot and with a fork, cushion the couscous.

0) Meanwhile, in a bowl, add the yogurt, lemon juice, remaining garlic and 2

tbsp. water and beat until well combined.

In the lower part of each serving plate, partition the yogurt sauce equitably and top with couscous, chicken cuts, cucumbers, tomatoes, Kalamata olives, feta and dill.

Drizzle with the excess olive oil and serve.

Nutrition Information:

Calories per serving: 808; Carbohydrates: 46.2g; Protein: 62.5g; Fat: 40.8g; Sugar: 7.8g; Sodium: 123mg; Fiber: 4.1g

17– Protein-Packed Bowl

6 people

Cooking Time: 6 minutes Preparation Time: 20 minutes

Ingredients:

For Tzatziki Sauce:

1 C. plain Greek yogurt

1 cucumber, stripped, cultivated and grated

1 tbsp. new dill weed ¾ tsp. prepared salt ¼ tsp. newly ground dark pepper

For Chicken Bowl:

1½ C. chicken broth 1 C. uncooked quinoa

1 lb. boneless chicken bosoms, cut into 7-8 pieces

2 tsp. Greek seasoning

To taste, season with salt and freshly ground dark pepper.

1 cucumber, quartered

1 C. grape tomatoes, halved

1 C. Kalamata olives

1 (15-oz.) can chickpeas, washed and drained

Instructions:

) For tzatziki sauce: in a bowl, add all fixings and blend until well combined.

) Refrigerate until using.

) In the pot of Instant Pot, place the stock and quinoa and mix to combine.

) Arrange the chicken bosoms on top and sprinkle with the Greek flavoring, salt and dark pepper.) Secure the cover and spot the strain valve to"Seal" position.) Select "Manual" and cook under "High Pressure" for around 6 minutes.

) Select "Drop" and cautiously do a"Speedy" release.) Remove the top and move the chicken and quinoa into serving bowls evenly.) Top with chickpeas, vegetables and tzatziki sauce evenly. 0) Serve hot.

Nutrition Information:

Calories per serving: 421; Carbohydrates: 44.4g; Protein: 34.2g; Fat: 11.6g; Sugar: 5.5g; Sodium: 340mg; Fiber: 6.8g

18– Colorful Chicken & Rice Platter

6 people

Cooking Time: 18 minutes Time to prepare: 15 minutes
Ingredients:

2 tbsp. extra virgin olive oil

1½ lb. bone-in, skin-on chicken thighs

Salt, to taste

1 red ringer pepper, cultivated and chopped ½ of onion, sliced 3 cloves garlic, minced

1 tsp. ground cumin

1 tsp. red bean stew pepper

1 tsp. dried oregano

½ tsp. ground white pepper

Pinch of red pepper flakes

1 lb. tomatoes, chopped 1½ C. chicken broth 1 C. long-grain rice

1 C. frozen peas, to some degree thawed

Instructions:

) Place the oil in Instant Pot and select"Sauté". Then, at that point, add the chicken thighs and cook for around 3 minutes for each side.

) With an opened spoon, move the chicken thighs onto a plate.

) In the pot, add the ringer pepper, onion, and garlic and cook for around 4-5 minutes.

) Stir in the tomatoes and chicken stock and bring to a boil.

) Select "Drop" and mix in the rice and top with the cooked chicken thighs.

) Secure the cover and spot the tension valve to"Seal" position.

) Select "Manual" and cook under "High Pressure" for around 12 minutes.) Select "Drop" and do a "Whiz" release.) Remove the top and mix in the peas.

0

) Immediately, secure the top for around 5 minutes before serving. Nutrition Information: Calories per serving: 427; Carbohydrates: 3g; Protein: 38.8g; Fat: 14g; Sugar: 4.9g; Sodium: 342mg; Fiber: 3.5g

---

Chapter Three

Tuscan Chicken Rice

Serves: 3

Cooking Time: 15 minutes Time to prepare: 15 minutes

Ingredients:

1 cup of rice

a cup of chicken broth, heated to a temperature of 112 degrees Fahrenheit

3 chicken breasts, boneless and skinless

1/3 cup pesto (basil)

12 C. marinated artichoke hearts in oil, sliced 12 C. sun-dried tomatoes in oil, strain

mozzarella cheese, 1 cup

1 tbsp. seasoning (Italian)

Instructions: Place the rice and chicken broth in the Instant Cooker pot.

) Arrange the chicken bosoms in a single layer over the rice.) Spread the pesto equally over each chicken bosom.

) Arrange the artichoke hearts on top, followed by 14 C. sun-dried tomatoes.

Sprinkle the Italian seasoning over the tomatoes, cheddar, and leftover sun-dried tomatoes.)

) Close the lid and set the tension valve to "Seal" mode.) Select "Manual" and cook for 15 minutes on "High Pressure.") Do a "Whiz" release after selecting "Drop."

) Remove the cap and combine the ingredients.

0) Serve immediately.

Information about nutrition:

471 calories per serving 55.8 g carbohydrates; 41.1 g protein; 7.8 g fat; 2 g sugar; 553 mg sodium; 3.2 g fiber

20– Favorite Chicken Pasta from Italy

6 people

Time to prepare: 10 minutes Time to prepare: 15 minutes Ingredients:

1 tbsp. extra virgin olive oil

12 cup chopped onion

1 tbsp. minced garlic 134 C. chicken broth

8 oz. penne pasta, uncooked

Tenderloins of 112 pound chicken, sliced into slices

1 tsp. seasoning (Italian)

To taste, season with salt and freshly ground Black pepper.

1 container tomato-based spaghetti sauce (24 oz.)

1 (8-oz.) cream cheese bundle

3 c. chopped fresh spinach 2-3 tbsp. cornstarch

3 tablespoons of water

6 tablespoons shredded parmesan cheddar

Instructions:

) Select "Sauté" in the Instant Pot and add the oil. After that, add the onion and simmer for about 3-4 minutes.

) Cook for about 1 minute after adding the garlic.

) Choose "Drop" and add the broth.

) Arrange the spaghetti in a single layer, followed by the chicken pieces.) Season with Italian seasoning, salt, and freshly ground black pepper.) Distribute the spaghetti sauce evenly on top, followed by the cream cheddar block.) Place the tension valve in the "Seal" position and secure the top.) Select "Manual" and cook for around 4 minutes at "High Pressure."

) Select "Drop" and perform a 5-minute "Whiz" discharge, followed by a 5-minute "Fast" release.

Meanwhile, dissolve cornstarch with water in a bowl.

Take the top off and toss in the spinach.

Add the cornstarch to the saucepan and whisk constantly.

Select "sauté" and cook for around 1 minute, continually combining. 4) Select "Drop" and serve immediately with cheese fixings.

Information about nutrition:

629 calories per serving; 42.2 grams of carbohydrates; 45.9 grams of protein; 29.9 grams of fat; 10.9 grams of sugar; 1023 milligrams of sodium; 3.5 grams of fiber

21– Flavorful Chuck Shoulder RED MEAT RECIPES

6 people

Time to prepare: 45 minutes Time to prepare: 15 minutes

Ingredients:

2 pound boneless meat toss cook, controlled and cut into 2" 3D squares across the grain

3 tbsp. flour (usually helpful)

12 teaspoon oregano, dry

To taste, season with salt and freshly ground Black pepper.

1 large onion, finely sliced

2 tablespoons extra-virgin olive oil 4 shallots, sliced

12 C. Medjool dates, pitted and diced 1 garlic clove, minced

12 cup beef stock 14 cup balsamic vinegar 14 cup red wine

Instructions:

) Combine the flour, oregano, salt, and dark pepper in a mixing bowl.) Place the meat blocks and flour mixture in a sealable plastic bag.) Seal the package and shake it to evenly distribute the contents.

) Select "Sauté" in the Instant Pot after adding the oil. Then, after that, add

Cook for 4-5 minutes with the meat mixture, onions, shallots, and garlic.

) Choose "Drop" and toss in the remaining ingredients.

) Place the strain valve in the "Seal" position and secure the lid.

) Select "Manual" and cook for around 40 minutes at "High Pressure."

) Select "Drop" and press the "Whiz" button.) Remove the top and serve immediately.

Information about nutrition:

408 calories per serving 18.9 grams of carbohydrates; 47.5 grams of protein; 14.3 grams of fat; 11.2 grams of sugar; 194 milligrams of sodium; 1.7 grams of fiber

Yummy Chuck (number 22) Roast

6 people

Time to cook: 1 hour and 10 minutes

Time to prepare: 15 minutes

Ingredients:

1 teaspoon sweetener

2 tsp. powdered red bean stew

1 tablespoon paprika

12 teaspoon cayenne pepper

1 tbsp cumin powder

1 tbsp. powdered onion

1 tsp. cinnamon powder

To taste, season with salt and freshly ground Black pepper.

3 pound toss broil, cut into large slices

3 slivered garlic cloves

1 tbsp. extra virgin olive oil

1 cup of beef broth

Instructions:) Mix the Swerve, tastes, salt, and dark pepper together in a small dish.) Cut small incisions into the roast with a sharp knife.) Evenly stuff the garlic bits into the broil cuts.

) Cut the food into 6 even pieces now.

) Evenly rub the zest mixture into each food lump.

) Select "Sauté" in the Instant Pot after adding the oil. Then, after that, add

Cook for about 8-10 minutes, or until the dish is thoroughly seared.) Choose "Drop" and add the broth.) Place the strain valve in the "Seal" position and secure the top.) Select "Manual" and cook for around 60 minutes at "High Pressure."

Make a "Whiz" release after selecting "Drop."

Remove the lid off the meal and place the pieces on a chopping board.

Serve each lump by cutting it into small pieces.

Information about nutrition:

531 calories per serving; 3.9 grams of carbohydrates; 76.3 grams of protein; 21.9 grams of fat; 1.5 grams of sugar; 316 milligrams of sodium; 0.9 grams of fiber

23– Delicious Beef for Dinner

3 people

Time to prepare: 35 minutes Time to prepare: 15 minutes

4 dates, hollowed out and soaked in warm water

4 tbsp. oil-soaked sun-dried tomatoes

1 pound hurl roast of hamburger

2 tbsp. extra virgin olive oil

1 tablespoon minced shallot

4 minced garlic cloves

1 teaspoon oregano, dry

1 tsp. thyme (dried)

To taste, season with salt and freshly ground Black pepper.

1 tablespoon balsamic vinaigrette

1 cup chicken broth 1 teaspoon grated lemon zest

Instructions:

) Puree the dates and sun-dried tomatoes in a food processor until smooth. Place the date puree in a separate dish and put it aside.

) Select "Sauté" in the Instant Pot after adding the oil. After that, add the shallot and garlic and sauté for another minute.) Add the meat to the pan and cook for about 2 minutes on each side.) Select "Drop" and stir in the other ingredients, except the lemon zest.) Place the strain valve in the "Seal" position and secure the top.) Select "Manual" and cook for 30 minutes on "High Pressure.") Select "Drop" and release "Whiz.") Remove the top of the meat and place it in a basin.) Shred the meat with two forks.

0

) Garnish with a zing of lemon and serve.

Information about nutrition:

705 calories per serving; 13.4 grams of carbohydrates; 42.3 grams of protein; 53.3 grams of fat; 7.4 grams of sugar; 428 milligrams of sodium; 1.9 grams of fiber

24– Zesty Italian Beef

8 people

Time to cook: 1 hour Time to prepare: 15 minutes Ingredients:

3 pound hurl cook hamburger, cut into huge pieces

gentle 12 (16-oz.) container Pepperoncini

1 (1 oz.) packet of spicy Italian dressing mix

1 teaspoon oregano, dry

1 tsp. basil (dried)

4 minced garlic cloves 1/3 cup Pepperoncini From the Jar: Juice

14 C. red wine 1 (1012 oz.) can pork broth

Instructions:

) Incorporate all of the ingredients in an Instant Pot pot and stir to combine.

) Place the strain valve in the "Seal" position and secure the top.) Select "Manual" and cook for around 60 minutes at "High Pressure.") Do a "Whiz" release after selecting "Drop.") Remove the top and place the meat in a basin.) Shred the hamburger with two forks and serve.

Information about nutrition:

648 calories per serving 4.2g carbohydrate; 45.5g protein; 47.7g fat; 0.2g sugar; 599mg sodium; 0.1g fiber

25– Meatballs for the Whole Family 5 Servings of Spaghetti

Time to cook: 11 minutes Time to prepare: 20 minutes Ingredients:

2/3 cup of water

1/3 cup quinoa, uncooked

1 pound of Italian sausage

2 finely minced garlic cloves

112 tsp oregano, dry

1 tsp. basil (dried)

12 tsp. parsley (dry)

granulated onion powder, 112 tsp

12 teaspoon salt

1 bottle tomato basil marinara sauce (24 oz.)

1 (12-oz.) spaghetti bundle

2 tbsp. basil leaves, chopped

Instructions:

) Place the quinoa and water in the Instant Pot pot.) Cover and set the strain valve to the "Seal" setting.) Select "Manual" and cook for 1 minute under "High Pressure.") Go to "Drop" and conduct a "Whiz" discharge for about 10 minutes, then go back to "Drop."

Do a "Speedy" release at that moment.

) Take the lid off the quinoa and place it in a bowl. Remove from the oven and set aside to cool somewhat.) Combine the quinoa, frankfurter, garlic, spices, oregano, onion powder, and salt in a mixing bowl and mix thoroughly with your hands.

) Form a 2-inch ball out of the mixture.) Place half of the marinara sauce in the bottom of the Instant Pot.) Place the meatballs on top of the sauce and drizzle with the remaining sauce. 0) Close the lid and set the tension valve to "Seal" mode. 1) Select "Manual" and cook for around 10 minutes at "High Pressure." 2) Meanwhile, boil the spaghetti for 8-10 minutes in a dish of finely salted bubbling water, or according to the package guidelines. 3) Flush the spaghetti under cold running water after draining it. 4) Arrange the pasta on individual serving dishes. 5) Select "Drop" on the Instant Pot and conduct a "Fast" release slowly. 6) Remove the lid and spoon the meatballs sauce over each dish of pasta.

17) Serve with basil as a garnish.

Information about nutrition:

669 calories per serving; 64.5 grams of carbohydrates; 29.6 grams of protein; 31.7 grams of fat; 12.3 grams of sugar; 1480 milligrams of sodium; 4.6 grams of fiber

26– Osso Buco Lombard

4 people

Time to cook: 1 hour and 33 minutes Time to prepare: 15 minutes Ingredients:

4 fresh sprigs of thyme

2 rosemary sprigs fresh

4 (10-oz.) bone-in veal knives, patted dry 1 straight leaf

To taste, season with salt and freshly ground Black pepper.

12 C. flour (all-purpose)

extra-virgin olive oil, 3 tbsp.

2 tbsp butter (unsalted)

2 large carrots, peeled and cut into 14-inch chunks

1 large onion, sliced into 14-inch chunks

1 celery stalk, sliced into 14-inch chunks

4 finely sliced garlic cloves

12 tablespoons tomato paste

12 oz. dry white wine, 12 oz.

12 c. chicken stock

1 can diced tomatoes (1412 oz.) drained

Tie the spice branches and straight leaves together with kitchen thread.) Season the veal knives with salt and black pepper, then cover them.

In the Instant Pot, choose "Sauté" and pour in the flour equally. Then, in two groups, add the knives and cook for about 5-7 minutes on each side.) Place the knife on a dish and add the margarine, carrot, onion, and celery to the saucepan, cooking for 6-8 minutes.) Stir in the garlic and tomato glue, and simmer for another 1-2 minutes.) Pour in the wine and scrape the bottom of the pan to remove the charred bits.) Choose "Drop" and add the broth.

) Place the spice bag on top of the cooked knives and submerge them in the vegetable mixture.

0) Tighten the top and set the tension valve to "Seal." 1) Select "Manual" and cook for around 40 minutes at "High Pressure." 2) Do a "Whiz" release after selecting "Drop."

3) Remove the lid and place the knife on a dish using an open spoon. 4) Select "Sauté" and simmer for 10-15 minutes, or until desired sauce thickness is achieved.

15) Select "Drop" and set aside the sauce for about 10 minutes. 16) Scrape any excess fat off the top with an open spoon. 17) Place the osso buco on a serving plate and pour the sauce over it. 18) Serve right away.

Information about nutrition:

816 calories per serving; 23.7 grams of carbohydrates; 93.4 grams of protein; 34.4 grams of fat; 5.9 grams of sugar; 472 milligrams of sodium; 3.2 grams of fiber

27– What is your favorite Greek dish? Dinner

10 people

Time to cook: 1 hour and 2 minutes Time to prepare: 15 minutes For lamb, combine the following ingredients in a large mixing bowl.

extra-virgin olive oil, 2 tbsp.

5 pound boneless leg of lamb 3 chopped garlic cloves 1 crushed straight leaf

1 tsp. marjoram (dried)

1 tsp. thyme (dried)

1 tsp. sage (dried)

1 tsp. ginger powder

12 tsp. powdered dark pepper 1 tsp. sea salt

2 C. beef stock

212-3 pound potatoes, peeled and sliced into 2-inch chunks

To make the gravy:

arrowroot powder, 2/3 tbsp

1/3 cup of water

Instructions:

) Select "Sauté" in the Instant Pot and add the oil. After that, add the leg of sheep and cook for about 4-5 minutes on each side.

) Choose "Drop" and add the garlic, spices, salt, dark pepper, and broth to the pan.

) Secure the cover and turn the strain valve to the "Seal" position.) Select "Manual" and cook for around 50 minutes at "High Pressure."

) Select "Drop" and do a "Fast" release with caution.

) Take the top off the potatoes and toss them in.

) Tighten the top and set the tension valve to "Seal."

) Select "Manual" and cook for around 10 minutes on "High Pressure.") Select "Drop" and conduct a careful "Speedy" release.

Remove the lid and transfer the potatoes and sheep meat to a serving plate using an open spoon.

Cover the fundamentals with a piece of foil to keep them warm.

To make the sauce, dissolve the arrowroot powder in water in a small basin. 3) In a mixing bowl, combine the arrowroot powder and water, pounding constantly. 4) Choose "Sauté" and cook for 1-2 minutes.

Cut the meat into the desired size pieces.

Serve the essentials on individual plates.

Serve with a dollop of sauce on top.

537 calories per serving; 19.2 grams of carbohydrates; 66.7 grams of protein; 19.8 grams of fat; 1.5 grams of sugar; 520 milligrams of sodium; 2.9 grams of fiber

Leg of Lamb with an Aromatic Flavor

8 people

Preparation Time: 15 minutes Cooking Time: 134 hours

Ingredients:

6-8 garlic cloves, chopped into slivers 1 (4-412 lb.) boneless leg of sheep, string network removed

2 tbsp. extra virgin olive oil

To taste, season with salt and freshly cracked black pepper.

a teaspoon of garlic powder

1 tablespoon paprika

1 onion, quartered and stripped

2 crushed garlic cloves

1 c. white wine (dry)

7–10 sprigs thyme

3 sprigs rosemary

1 sprig oregano

2 tsp oregano, dried

2 leaves of the inlet

14 C. new lemon juice 114 C. chicken broth

Cut small cuts into the leg of lamb with a sharp knife.) Stuff the garlic fragments evenly into the meat cuts.) Drizzle the sheep with 1 tbsp. olive oil and season with the salt and pepper.

paprika, garlic powder, salt, and pepper.) In the Instant Pot, select "Sauté" with the leftover oil. Then add the sheep and cook for approximately 4-5 minutes on each side.) Transfer the sheep to a platter using an open spoon.) Add the onion to the pot and cook for 3-4 minutes.) Add the crushed garlic cloves and cook for 1 minute.) Add wine and cook for around 1-2 minutes, scraping up the carmelized bits from the bottom.\s) Select "Drop" and mix in the leftover ingredients.

Place the leg of sheep in the pot, crease side down.

Secure the top and spot the tension valve to"Seal" position. 2) Select "Manual" and cook under "High Pressure" for around 90 minutes. 3) Select "Drop" and do a "Whiz" release.

4) Remove the cover and spot the sheep onto cutting load up for around 10 minutes.

Through a fine cross section sifter, strain the pot squeezes and skim any abundance fat.

Cut the leg of sheep into wanted measured cuts and serve close by container juices.

Information about nutrition:

Calories per serving: 496; Carbohydrates: 3.8g; Protein: 65g; Fat: 20.5g; Sugar: 1.2g; Sodium: 315mg; Fiber: 0.7g

Chapter Four

Garlicky Lamb Shoulder

6 people

Cooking Time: 55 minutes Preparation Time: 1 minutes

Ingredients:

2¼ lb. sheep shoulder without a joint

4 garlic cloves, sliced\s5-6 new thyme twigs, divided\s1 tbsp. honey

To taste, season with salt and freshly ground Black pepper.

1 C. water

3 entire garlic cloves, peeled

Instructions:\s) Season the sheep shoulder with salt and dark pepper.\s) Spread 4 thyme twigs and garlic cuts all around the sheep shoulder.) Drizzle the sheep shoulder with the honey.\s) Carefully roll the meat together to get thyme branches and garlic slices.) Tie the sheep shoulder roll with butcher's strings.\s) In the pot of Instant Pot, place water, entire garlic clovesremaining thyme sprigs.\s) Place the sheep shoulder roll in the water.\s) Secure the cover and spot the strain valve to"Seal" position.) Select "Manual" and cook under "High Pressure" for around 40 minutes. 0) Select "Drop" and do a "Whiz" discharge for around 10 minutes, then, at\s

that point, do a "Fast" release.

Meanwhile, preheat the stove to 430 F. Orchestrate a rack in oven.

Remove the top of Instant Pot and move sheep shoulder onto a broiling tray.

Remove the butcher's string and permit the shoulder to unroll naturally.

Then heat the sheep shoulder for around 10-15 minutes or until the meat is sautéed slightly.

Remove from broiler and spot the sheep shoulder onto a cutting load up for around 10 minutes.

With a sharp blade, cut the sheep shoulder into wanted measured cuts and serve.

Information about the food:

Calories per serving: 332; Carbohydrates: 4g; Protein: 48g; Fat: 12.5g; Sugar: 2.90g; Sodium: 158mg; Fiber: 0.1g

30– Spice Marinated Lamb Shanks

3 portions

Cooking Time: 56 minutes 15 minutes for preparation

Ingredients:\sFor Marinade Mixture:

¼ C. olive oil

3 garlic cloves, minced

2 tbsp. brown sugar

1 tbsp. dried oregano

1 tbsp. smoked paprika

½ tsp. ground cumin\s1 cinnamon stick

For Lamb Shanks:

3 sheep shanks\s¼ C. olive oil

3 carrots, stripped and chopped

1 onion, chopped\s2 narrows leaves

2 C. red wine

4 C. warm hamburger broth

3 tbsp. cornstarch

3 tbsp. cold water

¼ C. new Italian parsley, chopped

Instructions:

) For marinade: in an enormous bowl, add all fixings and blend until well combined.

) Add legs of lamb and coat with marinade generously.

) Set to the side at room temperature to marinate for somewhere around 30 minutes.

) Remove the legs of lamb from bowl, saving any excess marinade.\s) Select "Sauté" from the Instant Pot's menu. Then, at that point, add the legs of lamb and cook for around 3-4 minutes for every side.

) With an opened spoon, move the knifes onto a plate.\s) In the pot, add the carrots, onion, straight leaves and held marinade and cook for around 4-5 minutes.\s) Stir in the wine and cook for around 10 minutes.\s) Select "Drop" and spot the knifes and stock in the pot.

Secure the top and spot the tension valve to"Seal" position.

Choose "Manual" and cook for about 30 minutes at "High Pressure."

Do a "Whiz" release after selecting "Drop."

Remove the top and with an opened spoon, move the knifes onto a plate.

Strain the fluid and return to pot, disposing of solids.

In a little bowl, disintegrate the cornstarch in water.

In the pot, add the cornstarch blend, beating continuously.

Select "sauté" and cook for around 2-3 minutes, mixing continuously.

Select "Drop" and pour the sauce over shanks.

Serve immediately.

Information about the food:

Calories per serving: 965; Carbohydrates: 31.8g; Protein: 88g; Fat: 40g; Sugar: 12.9g; Sodium: 123mg; Fiber: 1.4g

31– Succulent Lamb Shanks

4 portions

Cooking Time: 1 hour 5 minutes 15 minutes for preparation
Ingredients:

4 (10-oz.) sheep shanks

To taste, season with salt and freshly ground black pepper.

2 tbsp olive oil (extra virgin)

12 oz. white wine (dry)

1 medium onion, quartered

2 garlic cloves, minced

1 enormous carrot, stripped and quartered

1 little fennel bulb, quartered, fronds reserved

1 cove leaf

2¼ C. chicken broth

8 oz. dried cannellini beans, splashed for 24 hours, depleted and rinsed   1 huge carrot, stripped and cleaved roughly\s1 medium tomato, cultivated and chopped

Instructions:\s) Season the legs of lamb with salt and dark pepper.\s) With a piece of foil, cover the knifes and put away at room temperature for 2 hours.\s

) Select "Sauté" from the Instant Pot's menu. Then, at that point, add the legs of lamb in 2 clumps and cook for around 3-4 minutes for every side.

) With an opened spoon, move the knifes onto a plate.

) In the pot, add the wine and cook for around 3-4 minutes, scraping up the carmelized bits from the bottom.\s) Select "Drop" and mix in the knifes, onion, quartered carrot, fennel, garlic and straight leaf.\s) Secure the top and spot the tension valve to "Seal" position.\s) Select "Manual" and cook under "High Pressure" for around 35 minutes.\s) Select "Drop" and do a "Whiz" discharge for around 10 minutes, then, at that point, do a "Fast" release.

Remove the cover and with an opened spoon, move the knifes onto a plate.

Strain the fluid and return to the skillet, disposing of the vegetables.

Add the beans, cleaved carrot and tomato and mix to combine.

Secure the top and spot the tension valve to"Seal" position.

Select "Manual" and cook under "High Pressure" for around 10 minutes.

Select "Drop" and do a "Whiz" discharge for around 10 minutes, then, at that point, do a "Speedy" release.

16) Remove the top and gap the beans blend into serving bowls. 17) Top each bowl with 1 knife and serve.

Information about the food:

Calories per serving: 733; Carbohydrates: 22.2g; Protein: 87g; Fat: 29g; Sugar: 5.4g; Sodium: 889mg; Fiber: 6.8g

32– Tomato Braised Lamb Shanks

4 portions

Cooking Time: 1 hour 5 minutes 15 minutes for preparation
Ingredients:

olive oil, 2 tbsp.

4 (1-lb.) sheep shanks

To taste, season with salt and freshly ground black pepper.

4 garlic cloves, minced\s¾ C. dry red wine

1 (28-oz.) can squashed tomatoes

1 tsp. dried basil\s¾ tsp. dried oregano

¼ C. new parsley, chopped

Instructions:\s) Season the legs of lamb with salt and dark pepper.\s) Select "Sauté" from the Instant Pot's menu. Then add

the legs of lamb in 2 clusters and cook for around 3-4 minutes for each side.\s

) With an opened spoon, move the knifes onto a plate.

) In the pot, add the garlic and cook for around 1 minute.

) Add the wine and cook for around 2-3 minutes, scraping up the sautéed bits from the bottom.\s) Stir in the tomatoes, basil and oregano and cook for around 2 minutes.

) Select "Drop" and spot the knifes in the pot.

) Place the strain valve in the "Seal" position and secure the top. Select "Manual" and cook under "High Pressure" for around 45 minutes.

Do a "Whiz" release after selecting "Drop."

Remove the top and serve hot.

Nutrition Information:\sCalories per serving: 999; Carbohydrates: 18.5g; Protein: 132.9g; Fat: 37.3g; Sugar: 11.5g; Sodium: 724mg; Fiber: 6.7g

33– Greek Flavoring Meatballs

4 portions

10 Minutes of Preparation 20 minutes of preparation time

Ingredients: For Meatballs:\s¼ C. panko breadcrumbs\s¼ C. milk

1 lb. ground lamb

1 tsp. ground coriander

1 tsp. ground cumin

1 garlic clove, minced

1 tblsp oregano (dried)

1 tbsp. new mint leaves, chopped

To taste, season with salt and freshly ground black pepper.

¼ C. feta cheddar, crumbled

1 tablespoon of extra virgin olive oil

For Salad:

1 head margarine lettuce, attacked pieces

1 huge tomato, chopped\s1 C. blended olives, pitted\s1 medium cucumber, meagerly sliced

For Tzatziki Sauce:\s¼ C. cultivated and diced cucumber

Salt, to taste

½ C. plain Greek yogurt

1 garlic clove, minced finely

1 tablespoon of extra virgin olive oil

¼ tsp. dried dill

Instructions:

) For meatballs: in an enormous bowl, add every one of the fixings with the exception of oil and blend until well combined.

) Make 1-inch balls from the mixture.

) Arrange the trivet in the lower part of Instant Pot and pour 1 C. of water.\s) Place the meatballs on top of trivet in a solitary layer.\s) Secure the top and spot the strain valve to"Seal" position.

) Select "Manual" and cook under "High Pressure" for around 5 minutes.

) Choose "Drop" and release "Fast" with caution.

) Remove the cover and move the meatballs onto a plate.\s) Remove the water and trivet from pot.

With paper towels, wipe off the pot completely.

Select "Sauté" from the Instant Pot's menu. Then, at that point, add the meatballs and cook for around 4-5 minutes or until seared completely. 12) Meanwhile, for salad: in a bowl, combine as one all ingredients. 13) For tzatziki sauce: in another bowl, add every one of the fixings and blend well.

Divide the plate of mixed greens onto serving plates.

Select "Drop" and separation the meatballs onto each plate. 16) Top with tzatziki sauce and serve.

Information about the food:

Calories per serving: 425; Carbohydrates: 14.5g; Protein: 37.4g; Fat: 22.6g; Sugar: 6.6g; Sodium: 561mg; Fiber: 2.9g

34– Abruzzi Style Lamb Pasta

6 portions

Cooking Time: 50 minutes 15 minutes for preparation

Ingredients:\s1½ lb. sheep flank chops

2 tbsp olive oil (extra virgin)

1 yellow onion, slashed finely

2 garlic cloves, minced

1/3 C. dry red wine

1 (24-oz.) container tomato basil sauce

1 tbsp. tomato paste

1/8 tsp. red pepper flakes

To taste, season with salt and freshly ground black pepper.

½ C. water

1 lb. pappardelle pasta

1/3 C. parmesan cheddar, shredded

Instructions:\s) Season the sheep slashes with salt and dark pepper evenly.) Place the oil in Instant Pot and\s

select"Sauté". Then add

the sheep cleaves and cook for around 2-3 minutes for every side.) With an opened spoon, move the sheep slashes onto a plate.) In the pot, add the onion and garlic and cook for around 4-5 minutes.) Add the wine and cook for around 3-4 minutes, scraping up the seared

pieces from the bottom.\s) Select "Drop" and mix in the sheep hacks, pureed tomatoes, tomato glue, red pepper chips, salt and dark pepper.\s) Secure the cover and spot the tension valve to"Seal" position.) Select "Manual" and cook under "High Pressure" for around 35 minutes.) Meanwhile, in a container of the gently salted bubbling water, cook the\spasta for around 8-10 minutes or as per bundle directions. 0) Drain the pasta for and flush under cool running water.

Divide the pasta onto serving plates.

Select "Drop" of Instant Pot and do a "Whiz" discharge for around 10 minutes, then, at that point, do a "Fast" release.

Remove the top and spot the lab blend over pasta onto each plate. 4) Top with cheddar and serve.

Nutrition Information:\sCalories per serving: 536; Carbohydrates: 50.6g; Protein: 44g; Fat: 16.2g; Sugar: 6g; Sodium: 807mg; Fiber: 2.2g

FISH & SEAFOOD RECIPES\s41– Simplest Frozen Salmon

Serves: 2

Cooking Time: 4 minutes Preparation Time: 10 minutes
Ingredients:

1 C. cold water

¼ C. new lemon juice

2 (5-6-oz.) frozen salmon fillets

Olive oil cooking spray

To taste, season with salt and freshly ground black pepper.

Instructions:

) Arrange the trivet in the lower part of Instant Pot and pour water and lemon juice.

) Spray the salmon filets with cooking shower evenly.

) Place the salmon filets on top of trivet in a solitary layer, skin-side down.

) Place the strain valve in the "Seal" position and secure the lid.

) Select "Steam" and simply utilize the default season of 3-4 minutes.

) Choose "Drop" and release "Fast" with caution.

) Remove the top and move the salmon filets onto a platter.\s) Sprinkle with salt and dark pepper and serve.

Information about the food:

Calories per serving: 232; Carbohydrates: 0.6g; Protein: 33.2g; Fat: 10.7g; Sugar: 0.6g; Sodium: 159mg; Fiber: 0.1g

42– Omega-3 Rich Salmon\sServes: 4

Cooking Time: 5 minutes Preparation Time: 10 minutes

Ingredients:\s4 (4-oz.) salmon fillets

To taste, season with salt and freshly ground black pepper.

1/3 C. new parsley, chopped\s1/3 C. scallions, chopped\s½ C. canned diced tomatoes with basil, garlic and oregano   1 lemon, cut into 4 slices

Instructions:\s) Arrange 4 bits of foil onto a smooth surface.\s

) Season every salmon filet with salt and dark pepper.\s) Place 1 salmon filet in the focal point of each foil piece and top each with parsley, trailed by scallion, tomatoes and 1 lemon slice) Wrap each foil piece around the salmon to get it.

) Arrange the trivet in the lower part of Instant Pot and pour 1 C. of water.) Place the salmon packages on top of trivet in a solitary layer.) Secure the top and spot the strain valve to "Seal" position.) Select "Steam" and simply utilize the default season of 5 minutes.) Select "Drop" and cautiously do a "Fast" release.

0

) Remove the cover and move the salmon bundles onto a platter. 1) Carefully, open each bundle and serve.

Information about the food:

Calories per serving: 160; Carbohydrates: 2.2g; Protein: 22.5g; Fat: 7.1g; Sugar: 0.9g; Sodium: 94mg; Fiber: 0.8g

43– Welcoming Salmon Dinner Serves: 4

Cooking Time: 3 minutes 15 minutes for preparation

Ingredients: ¼ C. olive oil

1 tbsp. red wine vinegar

1 tbsp. new lemon juice

1 tbsp. feta cheddar, crumbled

1 garlic clove, minced ¼ tsp. dried oregano

To taste, season with salt and freshly ground black pepper.

4 (4-oz.) new salmon fillets

2 fresh sprigs of rosemary

2 lemon slices

Instructions:

) For sauce: in a bowl, add the oil, vinegar, lemon juice, feta cheddar, garlic, oregano, salt and dark pepper and beat until well combined.) Season every salmon filet with a spot of salt and dark pepper.

) Arrange the trivet in the lower part of Instant Pot and pour 1 C. of water.) Arrange the trivet in the lower part of Instant Pot and pour 1 C. of water.) Place the salmon filets on top of trivet in a solitary layer.

) Secure the top and spot the tension valve to"Seal" position.

) Select "Manual" and cook under "High Pressure" for around 3 minutes.) Select "Drop" and cautiously do a"Fast" release.) Remove the cover and serve hot. Information about the food:

Calories per serving: 267; Carbohydrates: 0.5g; Protein: 22.4g; Fat: 20.1g; Sugar: 0.2g; Sodium: 116mg; Fiber: 0.1g

44– Flavor-Packed Cod

4 portions

Cooking Time: 8 minutes 15 minutes for preparation

Ingredients:

1 lb. cherry tomatoes, halved

2-3 new thyme sprigs

4 cod fillets

1 C. dark salt-restored Kalamata olives

2 tbsp. cured capers

2 tbsp. olive oil, divided

1 garlic clove, pressed

To taste, season with salt and freshly ground black pepper.

Instructions:

) Arrange the liner bushel in the lower part of Instant Pot and pour 2 C. of water.) Line the lower part of a hotness resistant bowl for certain cherry tomatoes, trailed by thyme sprigs.

) Arrange cod filets on top, trailed by the leftover cherry tomatoes, garlic.) Drizzle with 1 tbsp. of olive oil and sprinkle with a touch of salt and dark pepper.) Place the bowl in liner basket.

) Close the top and set the tension valve to "Seal."

) Select "Manual" and cook under "Low Pressure" for around 8 minutes.

) Select "Drop" and cautiously do a"Fast" release.) Remove the top and gap the cod filets and tomatoes onto the serving plates.

Top each filet with olives and escapades and sprinkle with some dark pepper.

Drizzle with residual oil and serve.

Nutrition Information: Calories per serving: 258; Carbohydrates: 7g; Protein: 31.8g; Fat: 12.4g; Sugar: 3g; Sodium: 571mg; Fiber: 2.6g

Chapter Five

One-Pot Dinner Cod

Serves: 2

Cooking Time: 5 minutes Preparation Time: 10 minutes
Ingredients:

2 (5-oz.) new cod fillets

¼ tsp. garlic powder

To taste, season with salt and freshly ground black pepper.

2 new dill sprigs

4 lemon slices

2 tsp. butter

1 C. water

Instructions:) Arrange 2 enormous square sheets of material paper onto a smooth surface.) Place 1 cod filet in the focal point of every material paper and sprinkle

with garlic powder, salt and dark pepper.) Top each filet with dill, trailed by lemon cuts and butter.) Wrap every material paper around the cod filet, passing on space for

steam to build.

) Arrange the trivet in the lower part of Instant Pot and pour 1 C. of water.) Place the cod bundles on top of trivet in a solitary layer.

) Close the lid and set the tension valve to "Seal.") Select "Manual" and cook under "High Pressure" for around 5 minutes.) Select "Drop" and cautiously do a "Fast" release.

0

) Remove the top and move the salmon packages onto a platter. 1) Carefully, open each package and serve.

Information about the food:

Calories per serving: 151; Carbohydrates: 0.8g; Protein: 25.5g; Fat: 25.5g; Sugar: 0.2g; Sodium: 197mg; Fiber: 0.2g

46– Terrific Protein Dinner

4 portions

Cooking Time: 4 minutes 15 minutes for preparation
Ingredients:

4 (4-oz.) frozen tilapia fillets

To taste, season with salt and freshly ground black pepper.

3 Roma tomatoes, chopped ¼ C. new basil, chopped 2 garlic cloves, minced 2 tbsp. olive oil

balsamic vinegar, 1 tblsp.

Instructions:) Season the tilapia filets with salt and dark pepper lightly.

) Arrange the trivet in the lower part of Instant Pot and pour ½ C. of water.) Place the cod

packages on top of trivet in a solitary layer.

) Place the strain valve in the "Seal" position and secure the lid.) Select "Manual" and cook under "High Pressure" for around 4 minutes.) Select "Drop" and cautiously do a "Speedy" release.

) Meanwhile, in a bowl, add the tomatoes, basil, garlic, oil, vinegar, salt

and dark pepper and throw to cover well.) Remove the top of Instant Pot and move the filets onto serving plates.) Top each filet with tomato blend and serve.

Information about the food:

Calories per serving: 173; Carbohydrates: 4.2g; Protein: 22.1g; Fat: 8.2g; Sugar: 2.5g; Sodium: 84mg; Fiber: 1.2g

47– Robust Fish Meal Serves: 4

Cooking Time: 4 minutes 15 minutes for preparation

Ingredients:

¼ C. water

4 (4-oz.) frozen ocean bass fillets

12 cherry tomatoes

12-14 dark olives

2 tbsp. marinated child capers

1/3 C. cut cooked red peppers

olive oil, 2 tbsp.

Salt, to taste

Pinch of red pepper flakes

Instructions:) In the pot of Instant Pot, pour the water.

) Place the fish filets in water and top with tomatoes, trailed by the olives, tricks and red peppers.

) Drizzle with olive oil and sprinkle with salt and red pepper flakes.

) Place the strain valve in the "Seal" position and secure the lid.

) Select "Manual" and cook under "High Pressure" for around 4 minutes.

) Select "Drop" and do a "Whiz" discharge for around 8 minutes, then, at that point, do a "Fast" release.

) Remove the top and move the fish blend onto serving plates.
) Serve hot.

Information about the food:

Calories per serving: 229; Carbohydrates: 3.8g; Protein: 27.6g; Fat: 11.5g; Sugar: 1.9g; Sodium: 419mg; Fiber: 1.3g

48– Tuna from the south of Italy Pasta serves 4 people.

Time to cook: 6 minutes Time to prepare: 15 minutes

12 oz. uncooked penne pasta Ingredients

2 C. halved cherry tomatoes 1/3 C. pitted and halved oil-restored olives

1 small sweet onion, thinly sliced

4 finely sliced garlic cloves

3 tbsp. extra virgin olive oil

a quarter teaspoon of red pepper flakes

To taste, season with salt and freshly ground Black pepper.

234°C water

1 fish steak (8 oz., 112-inch thick)

12 C. fresh basil leaves, chopped 112 tsp. coarsely ground lemon zing

2 tbsp. freshly squeezed lemon juice

Add the pasta, tomatoes, olives, onion, olives, garlic, oil, red pepper chips, salt, dark pepper, and water to the Instant Pot pot and stir to blend.

) Place the fish steak on top of the pasta mixture.) Close the lid and set the tension valve to "Seal.") Select "Manual" and cook for 6 minutes on "Low Pressure.") Choose"Drop" and execute a cautious"Speedy" release.

) Remove the top and stir in the basil, lemon zest, and lemon juice.) Cut the fish steak into smaller pieces and combine with the spaghetti sauce. Before serving, set aside for about 5 minutes.

Information about nutrition:

483 calories per serving; 53.8 grams of carbohydrates; 28 grams of protein; 17.5 grams of fat; 3.4 grams of sugar; 194 milligrams of sodium; 2 grams of fiber

56– Spring Side Dish VEGETARIAN & VEGAN RECIPES

5 people

Time to cook: 2 minutes Time to prepare: 10 minutes

Ingredients:

1 cup of ice cold water

Asparagus, 112 lb., trimmed

1 minced garlic clove

1 teaspoon of lemon zest

3 tbsp. extra virgin olive oil

1 tbsp. freshly squeezed lemon juice

To taste, season with salt and freshly ground Black pepper.

Instructions:

) Place the trivet in the bottom of the Instant Pot and fill with water.) Arrange the asparagus spears on the trivet.

) Go to "Steam" and choose the 0 minute season as the default.) Select "Drop" and do a "Fast" release with caution.

) Remove the lid from the asparagus and place it in a dish.

) Take the trivet and water out of the pot.

) Wipe the pot clean using paper towels.

) Select "Sauté" in the Instant Pot and add the oil. Then, after that, add

Cook for 1 minute with the garlic and lemon zing.) Cook for 1 minute after adding the cooked asparagus, lemon juice, salt, and dark pepper.

0) Choose "Drop" and serve right away.

Calories per serving: 101; Calories per serving: 101; Calories per serving: 101; Calories per serving 5.6g carbohydrate; 3.1g protein; 8.6g fat; 2.7g sugar; 34mg sodium; 2.9g fiber

57– Lunch with a Lot of Carbs

4 people

15-minute cooking time Time to prepare: 15 minutes Ingredients:

14 oz. chopped fresh spinach

4 medium potatoes, sliced into huge chunks 14 cup extra-virgin olive oil 1 cup water 2 tbsp. freshly squeezed lemon juice 4 chopped garlic cloves

To taste, season with salt and freshly ground Black pepper.

Instructions:

) Incorporate all of the ingredients in an Instant Pot pot and stir to combine.

) Place the strain valve in the "Seal" position and secure the top.) Select "Manual" and cook for 15 minutes on "High

Pressure.") Select "Drop" and conduct a "Fast" release with caution.) Remove the lid and serve.

284 calories per serving; 38.2 grams of carbohydrates; 6.7 grams of protein; 13.3 grams of fat; 3.1 grams of sugar; 134 milligrams of sodium; 7.4 grams of fiber

58– 3 Vegetables 6 people may be served with this combo.

Time to cook: 17 minutes Time to prepare: 20 minutes

Ingredients:

12 c. extra-virgin extra-virgin olive oil

2 quartered potatoes 1 pound fresh green beans, trimmed 1 big zucchini, quartered 112 onion, thinly sliced

1 can chopped tomatoes (15 oz.)

12 bundle fresh parsley, chopped 1 tsp. dried oregano 1 pack new dill, chopped

1 C. water, salt and freshly ground dark pepper to taste

Instructions:

) Select "Sauté" in the Instant Pot and add the oil. After that, toss in all of the veggies and simmer for around 1-2 minutes.

) Choose "Drop" and toss in the remaining ingredients.

) Place the strain valve in the "Seal" position and secure the lid.

) Select "Manual" and cook for 15 minutes on "High Pressure."
) Select "Drop" and make a careful "Speedy" release.) Remove the top and serve hot.

Information about nutrition:

251 calories per serving; 24.1 grams of carbohydrates; 4.3 grams of protein; 17.3 grams of fat; 5.9 grams of sugar; 47 milligrams of sodium; 6.5 grams of fiber

6 Servings 59– Winner Stuffed Acorn Squash

Time to prepare: 25 minutes Time to prepare: 20 minutes

12 CUP UNCOOKED WILD RICE INGREDIENTS

134°C water

season with salt to taste

3 (1-lb.) oak seed squashes, cut in half lengthwise, stems removed and

seeded

1 tbsp. extra virgin olive oil

12 tbsp. coarsely sliced yellow onion

8 oz. fresh mushrooms, chopped coarsely 1 tbsp. garlic, minced

12 tsp dark pepper, freshly ground

1/3 C. low-sugar dried cranberries 1 (15-oz.) can low-sodium chickpeas, cleaned and drained

14 CUP WALNUTS, CRUMBLED

1 tbsp. chopped fresh thyme leaves

Instructions:

) Combine rice, water, and a pinch of salt in an Instant Cooker pot.) Place the strain valve in the "Seal" position and secure the top.) Select "Manual" and cook for 15 minutes on "High Pressure.") Do a "Whiz" release after selecting "Drop."

) Remove the lid and transfer the rice to a dish.) Wipe the pot clean with paper towels.

) Place the liner crate in the bottom of the Instant Pot and pour 12 C. of water into it.

water.

) Place the squash sections, cut sides up, in the liner container.) Cover the container and turn the tension valve to the "Seal" position. 0) Select "Manual" and cook for 4 minutes on "High Pressure." 1) Cut the top off the squash and arrange the pieces on a large serving platter.

plate.

Select "Drop" and perform a 5-minute "Whiz" discharge, followed by a 5-minute "Fast" release.

Meanwhile, in a large pan over medium heat, heat the olive oil and sauté the onion for about 4 minutes.

Sauté for about 1 minute after adding the garlic. 7 minutes 5)5)

Cook for 2 minutes after adding the chickpeas, cranberries, walnuts, thyme, and cooked rice.

Fill each squash half with the hot filling and serve right away. Information about nutrition: 473 calories per serving; 80.6 grams of carbohydrates; 19.5 grams of protein; 11.2 grams of fat; 9.3 grams of sugar; 55 milligrams of sodium; 18.1 grams of fiber

60– Quinoa with Herbs of Provence

6 people

Time to cook: 14 minutes Time to prepare: 10 minutes
Ingredients:

2 C. quinoa, soaked in water for 60 minutes, then drained

avocado oil (1 tbsp.)

1 sliced onion 1 minced garlic clove

Vegetable broth (212 C)

To taste, season with salt and freshly ground Black pepper.

lemon zest (1 tbsp.)

1 tsp. rosemary (dried)

1 teaspoon oregano, dry

1 tsp. marjoram (dried)

Instructions:

) Select "Sauté" in the Instant Pot and add the oil. Then add the onion and cook for a further 8 minutes.

) Add the quinoa and garlic and simmer, stirring regularly, for about 5 minutes.

) Choose "Drop" and add the stock, salt, and dark pepper to taste.

) Place the strain valve in the "Seal" position and secure the lid.

) Select "Manual" and cook for 1 minute under "High Pressure."

) Choose "Drop" and do a "Whiz" discharge for around 10 minutes, followed by a "Speedy" release.

) Remove the lid and fluff the quinoa with a fork.) Serve warm.

238 calories per serving; 39.3 grams of carbohydrates; 10.4 grams of protein; 4.4 grams of fat; 1.1 grams of sugar; 349 milligrams of sodium; 4.8 grams of fiber

61– Vibrant Flavors 4 Servings of Loaded Meal

Cooking Time: not long

Preparation 15-minute time limit

1 C. washed quinoa 1 C. fresh shiitake mushroom, sliced 12 C. carrots, peeled and shredded 12 C. cherry tomatoes, split 14 C. hemp seeds, shelled 14 C. red onion, daintily sliced 14 C. black olives, pitted and chopped 1 small bunch of spinach

1 tbsp. extra virgin olive oil

To taste, season with salt and freshly ground Black pepper.

Instructions:

) Incorporate the stock, quinoa, and mushrooms in an Instant Pot pot and stir to combine.

) Tighten the top and set the tension valve to "Seal.") Select "Manual" and cook for 1 minute under "High Pressure.") Do a "Whiz" release after selecting "Drop."

) Take off the top and toss in the remaining ingredients.

) Set aside for about 5 minutes, covered, before serving.

RECIPES FOR SOUPS AND STEWS 71– Immunity-Boosting Chicken Soup

4 people

Time to prepare: 23 minutes Time to prepare: 15 minutes

Ingredients:

Mixture of Spices:

2 tsp. seasoning (Italian)

1 tablespoon turmeric

12 teaspoons garlic powder

14 tsp. cayenne pepper 14 tsp. ground ginger

Soup Ingredients:

1 pound boneless and skinless chicken bosoms, cubed

To taste, season with salt and freshly ground Black pepper.

1 tbsp. extra virgin olive oil

12 tbsp. finely sliced yellow onion

8 oz. kid carrots, halved 2 celery stems, cut

12 oz. cauliflower rice, frozen

8-12 oz. sliced frozen sweet potato

4 cup chicken stock

Instructions: To make the zest blend, put all of the ingredients in a mixing dish. Set aside.) Season the solid chicken forms equally with salt and black pepper. Select "Sauté" in the Instant Pot after adding the oil. Then, after that, add

Cook for around 2-3 minutes with the onion.

) Add the solid chicken forms and cook for 4-5 minutes.) Combine the flavors in a mixing bowl.

) Choose "Drop" and toss in the remaining ingredients.

) Tighten the top and set the tension valve to "Seal.") Select "Manual" and cook for 15 minutes on "High Pressure.") Select "Drop" and do a "Speedy" release with caution.

0) Remove the lid and serve immediately.

392 calories per serving; 23.9 grams of carbohydrates; 41.9 grams of protein; 14.3 grams of fat; 9.9 grams of sugar; 998 milligrams of sodium; 6.2 grams of fiber

72– Traditional Wedding Soup

10 people

Time to prepare: 10 minutes Time to prepare: 20 minutes

For Meatballs, combine the following ingredients in a large mixing bowl.

12 pound chicken sausage, ground

12 pound ground turkey 12 cup grated Parmesan cheese 14 cup milk

a single egg

1 sliced white bread, ripped

3 tsp. seasoning (Italian)

To taste, season with salt and freshly ground Black pepper.

12 teaspoons garlic powder

Soup Ingredients:

extra-virgin olive oil, 2 tbsp.

3 carrots, peeled and finely sliced

9 C. low-sodium chicken broth 2 celery stalks, chopped 1 big onion, diced 3 garlic cloves, minced

1 tsp. dill (dried)

34 C. pastina, salt and freshly ground black pepper to taste

10 oz. fresh spinach for kids

Instructions:

) To make meatballs, put all ingredients in a large mixing basin and mix well with your hands.

) Form the mixture into 1-inch meatballs.) Select "Sauté" in the Instant Pot after adding the oil. Then add the carrots, celery, and onion and simmer for 5-6 minutes.) After that, add the garlic and cook for 1 minute.) Choose "Drop" and add the stock, dill, salt, and dark pepper to taste.) Place the meatballs in the stock mixture carefully, followed by the pastina.) Place the tension valve in the "Seal" position and secure the top.) Select "Manual" and cook for 3 minutes on "High Pressure.") Select "Drop" and do a "Whiz" discharge for around 15 minutes, followed by a "Fast" discharge.

Take the top off and toss in the spinach.

Before serving, set the soup aside for about 5 minutes.

Information about nutrition:

256 calories per serving; 21.9 grams of carbohydrates; 18.8 grams of protein; 10.6 grams of fat; 2 grams of sugar; 312 milligrams of sodium; 1.4 grams of fiber

73– Soup with Pasta and Beans

8 people

Time to prepare: 27 minutes Time to prepare: 15 minutes

Ingredients:

1 tbsp. extra virgin olive oil

2 finely sliced celery stems

2 c. peeled and sliced carrots

4 garlic cloves, minced 1 large yellow onion, diced

112 pound ground beef

stew powder, 2 tsp

1 can chopped tomatoes (1412 oz.)

1 can (15 oz.) exceptional northern white beans, rinsed and drained 1 (15-oz.) can rinsed and drained red kidney beans

5 oz. elbow macaroni, uncooked

1 tomato sauce can (1412 oz.)

5 cup chicken stock

To taste, season with salt and freshly ground Black pepper.

12 C. grated Parmesan cheese

Instructions:

) Select "Sauté" in the Instant Pot and add the oil. Cook for another 4-5 minutes after that, adding the carrot, celery, and onion.

) Cook for about 1 minute after adding the garlic.

) Cook for 6-8 minutes after adding the ground hamburger.) Drain the oil from the saucepan.) Add the stew powder and cook for 1 minute.) Add the tomatoes and simmer for 6-8 minutes.

) Choose "Drop," then add the beans, pasta, pureed tomatoes, and broth.) Place the strain valve in the "Seal" position and secure the top.) Select "Manual" and cook for around 4 minutes at "High Pressure."

Select "Drop" and perform a 5-minute "Whiz" discharge, followed by a 5-minute "Fast" release.

Remove the top and serve with a cheese garnish.

Information about nutrition:

448 calories per serving; 46.3 grams of carbohydrates; 42 grams of protein; 10.4 grams of fat; 7.9 grams of sugar; 1203 milligrams of sodium; 11.8 grams of fiber

74– Rustic Tortellini Soup

8 people

Cooking Time: 21 minutes

Preparation Time: 5 minutes

Ingredients:\s1 lb. ground Italian sausage

1 medium white onion, chopped

2 garlic cloves, minced

1 (10-oz.) bundle frozen cheddar tortellini

1 enormous carrot, stripped and cut into ¼-inch rounds

1 (14-oz.) can modest diced tomatoes with juice

2 (8-oz.) jars tomato sauce

6 C. hamburger broth

1 inlet leaf

½ tsp. dried basil

12 teaspoon oregano, dry

1 medium zucchini, chopped

1 medium green chime pepper, cultivated and chopped

Instructions:

) Select "Sauté" in the Instant Pot and add the oil. Then, at that point, add the ground hotdog and cook for around 8-10 minutes, saying a final farewell to a wooden spoon.

) Drain off any abundance oil from the pot.\s) Add the onion and garlic and cook for around 4-5 minutes.

) Select "Drop" and mix in the tortellini, carrot, tomatoes, pureed tomatoes, stock, basil and oregano.\s) Secure the cover and spot the tension valve to"Seal" position.

) Select "Manual" and cook for 1 minute under "High Pressure."

) Select "Drop" and do a "Fast" release with caution.

) Remove the top and mix in the zucchini and chime pepper.\s) Select "Sauté" and cook for around 5 minutes.

Select "Drop" and dispose of the cove leaf.

Serve hot.

Information about nutrition:

Calories per serving: 318; Carbohydrates: 22.8g; Protein: 19.2g; Fat: 16g; Sugar: 8.4g; Sodium: 1400mg; Fiber: 2.8g

Chapter Six

Effortless Veggie Soup

6 people

15-minute cooking time Time to prepare: 15 minutes
Ingredients:

3 C. green cabbage, cleaved roughly\s2½ C. vegetable broth

1 can chopped tomatoes (1412 oz.)

3 carrots, stripped and chopped\s3 celery stems, chopped\s1 onion, chopped\s2 garlic cloves, chopped\s2 tbsp. apple juice vinegar

1 tbsp. freshly squeezed lemon juice

2 tsp. dried sage

Instructions:

) Incorporate all of the ingredients in an Instant Pot pot and stir to combine.

) Tighten the top and set the tension valve to "Seal.") Select "Manual" and cook for 15 minutes on "High Pressure.") Select "Drop" and do a "Whiz" release.\s) Remove the cover and serve hot.

Nutrition Information:\sCalories per serving: 62; Carbohydrates: 10.6g; Protein: 3.7g; Fat: 0.8g; Sugar: 5.7g; Sodium: 357mg; Fiber: 3.1g

76– Bright Green Soup

4 people

Cooking Time: 7 minutes Time to prepare: 15 minutes

Ingredients:

2 tbsp. extra virgin olive oil

1 huge celery stem, chopped\s1 medium onion, slashed finely

1 lb. broccoli, chopped\s2 medium white potatoes, stripped and cubed\s2 huge garlic cloves, chopped\s4 C. vegetable broth

To taste, season with salt and freshly ground Black pepper.

½ C. coconut cream

1 tbsp. freshly squeezed lemon juice

Instructions:

) Select "Sauté" in the Instant Pot and add the oil. Then, at that point, add the celery and onion and cook for around 3-4 minutes.

) Select "Drop" and mix in the leftover fixings aside from lemon juice.

) Secure the top and spot the tension valve to"Seal" position.\s) Select "Manual" and cook under "High Pressure" for around 3 minutes.\s) Select "Drop" and do a "Whiz" discharge for around 5 minutes, then, at that point, do a "Speedy" release.) Remove the top and with an inundation blender, mix the soup until smooth.\s) Stir in the coconut cream and lemon juice and serve.

Information about nutrition:

Calories per serving: 294; Carbohydrates: 30.1g; Protein: 11g; Fat: 16.1g; Sugar: 6.2g; Sodium: 856mg; Fiber: 6.9g

82– Sweet & Savory Stew

8 people

Time to cook: 1 hour Time to prepare: 15 minutes Ingredients:

3 tbsp. extra virgin olive oil

1½ onions, minced\s3 lb. hamburger stew meat, cubed\s1½ tsp. ground cinnamon

¾ tsp. paprika

¾ tsp. ground turmeric\s¼ tsp. ground allspice

¼ tsp. ground ginger

1½ C. meat broth\s1½ tbsp. honey

1½ C. dried apricots, split and absorbed high temp water until

mellowed and drained\s1/3 C. almond fragments, toasted\sInstructions:

) Place the oil in Instant Pot and select "Sauté". Then add theonion and cook for about 3-4 minutes.\s) Stir in the hamburger and cook for around 3-4 minutes or until sautéed completely.

Stir in the flavors and cook for around 2 minutes.

Select "Drop" and mix in the stock and honey.

Secure the cover and spot the strain valve to"Seal" position. 6) Select "Meat/Stew" and simply utilize the default season of 50 minutes. 7) Select "Drop" and do a "Whiz" discharge for around 15 minutes, then, at that point, do a "Speedy" release.

Remove the top and mix in the apricot halves.

Serve with the fixing of almond slivers.

Information about nutrition:

Calories per serving: 428; Carbohydrates: 10.1g; Protein: 54g; Fat: 18.4g; Sugar: 7.1g; Sodium: 257mg; Fiber: 1.9g

83– Wednesday Night Dinner Stew

6 people

Time to prepare: 35 minutes Time to prepare: 15 minutes

Ingredients:\s1½ lb. hamburger stew meat, managed and cut into 2-inch chunks   2 tbsp. olive oil

2 medium onions, chopped

2 garlic cloves, minced\s¼ C. tomato paste

4 C. meat broth

1½ C. dried split peas, rinsed

1 (28-oz.) can squashed tomatoes

1 tbsp cumin powder

½ tsp. saffron strings, crumbled

½ tsp. ground turmeric

¼ tsp. ground cinnamon

¼ tsp. ground allspice

To taste, season with salt and freshly ground Black pepper.

4 tbsp. new lemon juice

Instructions:\s) Season the hamburger lumps with salt and dark pepper evenly.) Select "Sauté" in the Instant Pot after adding the oil. Then, after that, add

the hamburger lumps in 2 bunches and cook for around 4-5 minutes or until carmelized completely.\s) With an opened spoon, move the meat pieces into a bowl.\s) In the pot, add the onions and garlic and cook for around 2-3 minutes.\s) Add the tomato glue and cook for around 1 minute.\s) Add the stock and cook for around 1 moment, scraping up any sautéed bits from the bottom.\s) Select "Drop" and mix in the cooked hamburger, split peas, tomatoes, flavors, salt and dark pepper.\s) Place the strain valve in the "Seal" position and secure the top.) Select "Manual" and cook under "High Pressure" for around 25 minutes.

Select "Drop" and do a "Whiz" discharge for around 15 minutes, followed by a "Fast" discharge.

Remove the top and mix in the lemon juice.

Serve hot.

Information about nutrition:

Calories per serving: 530; Carbohydrates: 47.7g; Protein: 54.1g; Fat: 13.7g; Sugar: 14.9g; Sodium: 888mg; Fiber: 18.3g

84– Comfy Meal Stew

6 people

Cooking Time: 1 hour 6 minutes Time to prepare: 15 minutes

Ingredients:\s¼ C. flour

To taste, season with salt and freshly ground Black pepper.

2 lb. sheep shoulder, cut into 1-inch cubes

2 tbsp. extra virgin olive oil

½ C. celery, chopped\s½ C. carrots, stripped and chopped\s½ C. fennel, chopped\s½ C. leeks, sliced\s1 tsp. dried rosemary, crushed\s2 tbsp. brandy

1 (28-oz.) can diced tomatoes

1 (15-oz.) can chickpeas, depleted and rinsed

2 C. beef stock

1 sound leaf\s2 tbsp. new parsley, chopped

Instructions:

) In a huge shallow bowl, combine as one the flour, salt and dark pepper.) Add the sheep 3D shapes and throw to cover well.\s) Select "Sauté" in the Instant Pot after adding the oil. Then, after that, add

the sheep 3D squares in 2 groups and cook for around 4-5 minutes.) With an opened spoon, move the sheep solid shapes into a bowl.) In the pot, add the celery, carrots, fennel and cook for around 5 minutes.) Stir in the rosemary and liquor and cook for around 1 moment, scraping up any seared pieces from the bottom.\s) Select "Drop" and mix in the cooked sheep blocks, tomatoes, chickpeas, stock and narrows leaf.\s) Place the strain valve in the "Seal" position and secure the top.) Select "Manual" and cook under "High Pressure" for around 45 minutes. 0) Select "Drop" and do a "Whiz" release.

1) Remove the top and serve hot with the embellishing of parsley. Information about nutrition: Calories per serving: 478; Carbohydrates: 28.5g; Protein: 49.7g; Fat: 17.4g; Sugar: 4.6g; Sodium: 634mg; Fiber: 5.7g

DESSERT RECIPES\s91– Berry Season Compote

8 people

Time to cook: 2 minutes Time to prepare: 10 minutes Ingredients:

4 C. new blended berries (strawberries, raspberries, blueberries and blackberries) (strawberries, raspberries, blueberries and blackberries)

¼ C. sugar

1 tsp. new lemon juice

1 tsp. squeezed orange concentrate

Instructions:

) In the pot of Instant Pot, place the berries and sugar and with a wooden spoon, mix until sugar is dissolved.

) Add the lemon juice and squeezed orange concentrate and mix to combine.

) Tighten the top and set the tension valve to "Seal."

) Select "Manual" and cook under "High Pressure" for around 2 minutes.

) Select "Drop" and do a "Whiz" discharge for around 10 minutes, then, at that point, do a "Speedy" release.\s) Remove the cover and let the blend cool before serving.

Nutrition Information:\sCalories per serving: 64; Carbohydrates: 14.8g; Protein: 0.5g; Fat: 0.3g; Sugar: 11.3g; Sodium: 0mg; Fiber: 2.5g

92– Elegant Dessert Pears\sServes: 6

Cooking Time: 13 minutes Time to prepare: 15 minutes Ingredients:

1 lemon, cut in half

3 C. water\s2 C. white wine

2 C. natural stick sugar

6 cinnamon sticks

6 ready, yet firm pears

9 oz. mixed chocolate, cut in ½-inch pieces

½ C. coconut milk

¼ C. coconut oil

2 tbsp. maple syrup

Instructions:

) Select "Sauté" of Instant Pot. Then, at that point, add the water, wine, sugar and cinnamon sticks and heat to the point of boiling, blending continuously.

) Meanwhile, strip the pears, keeping them entire, with the stems intact.) Immediately, rub every pear with lemon.

) Select "Drop" and get the excess lemon juice into the sugar syrup.) Place the squeezed lemon into the syrup.\s) Now, place the pears into the hot syrup.

) Place the strain valve in the "Seal" position and secure the lid.) Select "Manual" and cook under "High Pressure" for around 3 minutes.) Select "Drop" and cautiously do a"Fast" release.

0

) Remove the top and with an opened spoon, move the pears onto a platter. 1) Let the syrup cool slightly.

Place the cooled syrup over pears.

For chocolate sauce: place the chocolate in a bowl. Set aside.
4) In a little pan, place the coconut milk, coconut oil and maple syrup over

medium hotness and bring to a delicate simmer.

Remove from the hotness and promptly, pour the milk blend over the chocolate.

Let it sit for around 1 minute.

With a wire whisk, beat until smooth.

Pour the warm sauce over the pears and serve.

Information about nutrition:

Calories per serving: 712; Carbohydrates: 126.5g; Protein: 2.7g; Fat: 18.4g; Sugar: 45.5g; Sodium: 49mg; Fiber: 7g

93– Apple Juice Poached Pears

4 people

Time to cook: 6 minutes Time to prepare: 10 minutes

Ingredients:\s4 firm pears

4 C. unsweetened apple juice

1 C. frozen blackberries

2 cinnamon sticks

2 star anise

5 cardamom pods

2 tsp. vanilla extract\s

Instructions:\s) Peel pears and cut bottoms of pears, so they sit flat.\s) In the pot of Instant Pot, organize the pears, stem up and finish off

with apple juice.

) Submerge the blackberries, entire flavors and vanilla concentrate into the juice.

) Close the lid and set the tension valve to "Seal" mode.) Select "Manual" and cook under "High Pressure" for around 6 minutes.) Select "Drop" and do a "Fast" release with caution.

) Remove the top and with an opened spoon, move the pears onto a platter.) Through a fine cross section sifter, strain the juice,\s) Pour the juice over pears and serve.

Information about nutrition:

Calories per serving: 259; Carbohydrates: 64.5g; Protein: 1.4g; Fat: 0.7g; Sugar: 9.4g; Sodium: 11mg; Fiber: 8.6g

94– Chocolate Lover's Cake\sServe: 1

Time to prepare: 10 minutes Time to prepare: 15 minutes

Ingredients:\s4 tbsp. generally useful flour

4 tbsp. sugar

1 tbsp. cocoa powder

¼ tsp. orange zing, grated

Pinch of salt

½ tsp. baking powder

1 medium egg

4 tbsp. milk

extra-virgin olive oil, 2 tbsp.

Instructions:

) In a bowl, add all fixings and beat energetically until well combined.) Place the blend into a delicately lubed mug.

) Arrange the trivet in the lower part of Instant Pot and pour 1 cup of water.) Place the mug on top of the trivet.

) Place the strain valve in the "Seal" position and secure the lid.) Select "Manual" and cook under "High Pressure" for around 10 minutes.) Select "Drop" and do a "Speedy" release with caution.

) Remove the top and serve immediately.

Information about nutrition:

Calories per serving: 642; Carbohydrates: 79.50g; Protein: 11.8g; Fat: 34.7g; Sugar: 1.3g; Sodium: 249mg; Fiber: 2.6g

95– Moist Date Cake

Serves: 16

Cooking Time: 40 minutes Time to prepare: 20 minutes

Ingredients:\s1½ C. seedless dates, chopped\s1½ C. water\s1 tsp. baking soda

2 huge eggs\s¾ C. sugar\s½ C. unsalted spread, softened

1 tsp. vanilla extract

1½ C. generally useful flour\s¼ tsp. salt\s2 tsp. baking powder

1 tsp. moment espresso granules

1 tsp. unsweetened cocoa powder

Instructions:

) Select"Sauté" of Instant Pot and change it to the"More" mode. Then, at that point, add 1½ C. of water and bring to a boil.

) Add the dates and cook for around 5 minutes.

) Stir in the baking pop and select"Cancel".\s) Carefully eliminate the steel embed from the Instant Pot and put away for 15 minutes.\s) In a blender, add the eggs, sugar, spread and vanilla concentrate and heartbeat until well combined.

) Add the date combination and blend until well combined.

) Add the excess fixings and heartbeat until just combined.\s) Place the combination into a lubed 6-inch Bundt cake container evenly.\s) With a piece of foil, cover the pan.

Arrange the trivet in the lower part of Instant Pot and pour 1 C. of water.

Place the cake dish on top of the trivet.

Secure the top and spot the tension valve to"Seal" position.

Select "Manual" and cook for 30 minutes on "High Pressure."

Select "Drop" and do a "Whiz" discharge for around 15 minutes, followed by a "Fast" discharge.

15) Remove the cover and cautiously, move the Bundt skillet onto a wire rack. 16) Uncover the container and let it cool for around 10 minutes. 17) Carefully modify the cake onto the wire rack to cool totally before serving.

18) Cut the cake into wanted measured cuts and serve.

Information about nutrition:

Calories per serving: 186; Carbohydrates: 31.3g; Protein: 2.5g; Fat: 6.6g; Sugar: 20.1g; Sodium: 166mg; Fiber: 1.7g\s

96– Delicious Coffee-Time Cake

8 people

Time to prepare: 35 minutes Time to prepare: 15 minutes

Ingredients:\s2 C. generally useful flour

1 tsp. baking soda

1 tsp. baking powder

¼ tsp. salt

1 huge egg

1 C. plain unsweetened Greek yogurt

1 C. granulated sugar

½ C. unsalted spread, softened

3 tbsp. new lemon juice, divided\s1 tbsp. lemon zing, grated

1 C. confectioner's sugar

1 tbsp. half-and-half

Instructions:\s) In a bowl, combine as one the flour, baking pop, baking powder and salt.) In another bowl, add the egg, yogurt, granulated sugar, margarine, 2

tbsp. of lemon juice and lemon zing and with a hand blender, beat until smooth.\s) Add the flour combination and with the hand blender, blend until well combined.\s) Place the combination onto a lubed 6-C. Bundt dish evenly.\s) Arrange a paper towel over the highest point of container, then, at that point, cover the paper towel and skillet with a piece of foil loosely.\s) Arrange the trivet in the lower part of Instant Pot and pour 1 C. of water.\s) Place the cake dish on top of the trivet.\s) Secure the cover and spot the strain valve to"Seal" position.\s) Select "Manual" and cook under "High Pressure" for around 35 minutes.

Make a "Whiz" release after selecting "Drop."

Remove the top and cautiously, move the Bundt skillet onto a wire rack.

Uncover the container and let it cool for around 10 minutes.

Carefully modify the cake onto the wire rack to cool totally before glazing.

For glaze: in a bowl, add the confectioners' sugar, cream and remaining lemon squeeze and beat until smooth.

15) Spread the frosting over cake and serve.

Information about nutrition:

Calories per serving: 403; Carbohydrates: 66.7g; Protein: 6g; Fat: 13.1g; Sugar: 42.2g; Sodium: 348mg; Fiber: 0.9g

97– Delightful Cream Cake\s

Serves: 12

Time to prepare: 35 minutes Time to prepare: 15 minutes

Ingredients:\sFor Cake:

1 C. sharp cream

1 tsp. baking soda

1 C. butter

2 C. Turn confectioners

5 eggs

2½ C. whitened almond flour

1 C. unsweetened chipped coconut

1 tsp. baking powder

2 tsp. vanilla extract

For Frosting:

8 oz. cream cheddar, softened\s½ C. spread, softened\s1 tsp. vanilla extract\s2 C. Turn confectioners\s2 tbsp. weighty cream

½ C. pecans, chopped\s1 C. unsweetened chipped coconut

Instructions:

) Line the lower part of a lubed 7-inch round spring-structure cake dish with lubed material paper. Set aside.\s) For cake: in a little bowl, add the acrid cream and baking pop and blend well. Set aside.

) In a huge bowl, add margarine and sugar and beat until light and fluffy.\s) Add the leftover fixings and blend until just combined.\s) Place the combination into the pre-arranged cake skillet evenly.

) Arrange the trivet in the lower part of Instant Pot and pour 1 C. of water.\s) Place the cake dish on top of the trivet.\s) Secure the top and spot the tension valve to"Seal" position.\s)

Select "Manual" and cook under "High Pressure" for around 35 minutes.

0

) Select"Drop" and do a "Whiz" discharge for around 20 minutes, then, at that point, do a "Fast" release.

Remove the cover and cautiously, move the Bundt skillet onto a wire rack to cool for around 10 minutes.

Carefully modify the cake onto the wire rack to cool totally before frosting.

For frosting: in a medium bowl, add all fixings aside from pecans and chipped coconut and beat until light and fluffy.

Fold in the pecans and chipped coconut.

Spread the frosting over cake and serve.

Information about nutrition:

Calories per serving: 579; Carbohydrates: 9.2g; Protein: 6.3g; Fat: 56.4g; Sugar: 2g; Sodium: 363mg; Fiber: 4.1g